Prebiotics Health Guide for Beginners

Best Practices for Prebiotics Health

By

Baylen Angus

Table of Contents

CHAPTER 1

Introduction

1.1 What are Prebiotics

Prebiotics are non-digestible fibers and compounds found in certain foods that serve as a food source for beneficial gut bacteria. They are distinct from probiotics, which are live bacteria that confer health benefits when ingested in adequate amounts. Prebiotics, on the other hand, do not contain live bacteria themselves but instead act as nourishment for probiotics and other beneficial microorganisms residing in the gut.

The concept of prebiotics was first introduced by Dr. Marcel Roberfroid in 1995. He defined prebiotics as "non-viable food components that confer a health benefit on the host associated with modulation of the microbiota." In simpler terms, prebiotics are dietary compounds that promote the growth and activity of beneficial gut bacteria, leading to a healthier and more balanced gut microbiome.

The primary function of prebiotics is to selectively stimulate the growth and activity of beneficial bacteria, such as Bifidobacteria and Lactobacilli, while inhibiting the growth of harmful or pathogenic bacteria. When prebiotics reach the colon undigested, they become available as a nutrient source for these beneficial bacteria, helping them thrive and multiply.

Common types of prebiotics include:

1. Inulin: Found in foods like chicory root, Jerusalem artichoke, and dandelion greens, inulin is a type of soluble fiber that acts as a prebiotic by promoting the growth of beneficial bacteria in the colon.

2. Fructooligosaccharides (FOS): Present in foods such as garlic, onions, and bananas, FOS is another type of prebiotic that supports the proliferation of beneficial gut bacteria.

3. Galactooligosaccharides (GOS): These prebiotics are found in human breast milk and are added to some infant formulas. They promote the growth of beneficial Bifidobacteria in the infant gut.

4. Resistant Starch: Resistant starch is a type of starch that resists digestion in the small intestine and

reaches the colon intact. Foods rich in resistant starch, such as green bananas and cooked-and-cooled potatoes, serve as prebiotic compounds.

Prebiotics not only support gut health but also have far-reaching effects on overall health and well-being. As the gut microbiome plays a crucial role in various bodily functions, prebiotics indirectly impact immune function, nutrient absorption, metabolism, and even mental health.

Prebiotics are a class of non-digestible fibers and compounds found in specific foods that support the growth of beneficial gut bacteria. By nourishing these beneficial microorganisms, prebiotics contribute to a balanced and healthy gut microbiome, which in turn has positive effects on overall health.

Understanding the importance of prebiotics and incorporating them into our diets can be a fundamental step towards enhancing our well-being and optimizing our health journey.

1.2 The Importance of Gut Health

The human gut is a complex ecosystem that houses trillions of microorganisms, collectively known as the gut microbiome. This microbiome consists of various beneficial bacteria, viruses, fungi, and other microbes that play a crucial role in maintaining overall health. The importance of gut health extends far beyond just digestion; it influences numerous physiological processes and is now recognized as a central player in the interconnections between the gut, the brain, and other systems in the body.

Some key aspects of the importance of gut health include:

1. Digestion and Nutrient Absorption: The gut is responsible for breaking down and absorbing nutrients from the food we eat. A healthy gut with a diverse microbiome ensures efficient digestion and maximizes nutrient absorption, leading to better nourishment for the body.

2. Immune System Support: The gut plays a significant role in supporting the immune system. The gut-associated lymphoid tissue (GALT) houses immune cells that protect against harmful pathogens while maintaining tolerance to beneficial microbes. A balanced

gut microbiome helps regulate immune responses and reduces the risk of autoimmune disorders.

3. Mental Health and Mood Regulation: The gut and brain communicate through the gut-brain axis, a bidirectional communication system. The gut microbiome produces neurotransmitters and communicates with the brain, influencing mood, stress responses, and cognitive function. An imbalance in the gut microbiome has been linked to conditions like anxiety, depression, and other mental health issues.

4. Weight Management and Metabolism: Emerging research suggests that the gut microbiome may play a role in weight management and metabolic health.

An imbalanced gut microbiome has been associated with obesity and metabolic disorders.

5. Inflammatory Response: A healthy gut microbiome helps regulate inflammation in the body. Dysbiosis (an imbalance in gut bacteria) can lead to chronic inflammation, which is associated with various chronic diseases, including inflammatory bowel diseases (IBD), cardiovascular diseases, and certain cancers.

6. Regulation of Hormones: The gut microbiome can influence hormone regulation, impacting appetite, satiety, and metabolism.

Given the broad impact of gut health on overall well-being, maintaining a balanced and diverse gut microbiome is essential. This is where prebiotics come into play.

1.3 How Prebiotics Support Gut Health

Prebiotics play a pivotal role in supporting gut health by nourishing and promoting the growth of beneficial gut bacteria. When consumed, prebiotics pass through the upper digestive tract without being broken down or absorbed. They reach the colon mostly intact, where they serve as a food source for specific strains of beneficial bacteria, particularly Bifidobacteria and Lactobacilli.

As these beneficial bacteria feed on prebiotics, they ferment them into short-chain fatty acids (SCFAs), such as butyrate, acetate, and propionate.

SCFAs are essential for gut health and have multiple benefits, including:

1. Providing Energy for Colon Cells: SCFAs serve as an energy source for the cells lining the colon, supporting their health and integrity.

2. Maintaining Gut Barrier Function: SCFAs help strengthen the gut barrier, preventing the entry of harmful substances and pathogens into the bloodstream.

3. Modulating Immune Responses: SCFAs regulate the immune system, promoting a balanced response and reducing inflammation.

4. Regulating pH Levels: SCFAs help maintain a slightly acidic environment in the colon, which is beneficial for the growth of

beneficial bacteria and inhibitory to harmful ones.

By promoting the growth of beneficial bacteria and producing SCFAs, prebiotics help create a favorable environment in the gut that supports optimal digestion, immune function, and overall health. Regular consumption of prebiotic-rich foods can lead to a healthier and more diverse gut microbiome, which, in turn, can positively impact various aspects of well-being.

Understanding the significance of gut health is vital for overall wellness, as the gut microbiome influences digestion, immunity, mental health, metabolism, and various other physiological processes. Prebiotics play a critical role in supporting gut health by nourishing beneficial gut bacteria, which, in turn, produce essential short-chain fatty acids and contribute to a balanced and thriving gut ecosystem. Incorporating prebiotic-rich foods into our diets is a proactive step towards maintaining gut health and promoting overall well-being.

CHAPTER 2

Understanding the Gut Microbiome

2.1 The Microbiome: An Overview

The human body is home to a vast and diverse community of microorganisms, collectively known as the microbiome. Among the many microbiomes that exist within the body, the gut microbiome is one of the most complex and significant. It refers to the community of microorganisms residing in the gastrointestinal tract, primarily in the large intestine or colon.

The gut microbiome is composed of trillions of microbes, including bacteria, viruses, fungi, archaea, and other single-celled organisms. These microbes coexist in a delicate balance, forming a dynamic ecosystem that interacts with the host's body in numerous ways. The collective genetic material of these microorganisms significantly exceeds the number of human genes, making the microbiome an essential player in human health and disease.

The composition of the gut microbiome varies from person to person and can be influenced by various factors, including genetics, age, diet, environment, lifestyle, and medical history. Early-life factors, such as birth method (vaginal vs. cesarean), breastfeeding, and exposure to antibiotics, also play a crucial role in shaping the gut microbiome during infancy.

Functions of the Gut Microbiome:

1. Digestion: The gut microbiome assists in the digestion of certain dietary components that the human body cannot break down on its own. For example, microbes help break down complex carbohydrates, fiber, and other compounds into simpler molecules that the body can absorb and utilize for energy and other metabolic processes.

2. Nutrient Production: Some gut bacteria are capable of producing certain vitamins (e.g., B vitamins and vitamin K) and other essential nutrients, which can be absorbed and utilized by the host.

3. Immune System Regulation: The gut microbiome plays a significant role in educating and regulating the immune system. It helps the immune system differentiate between beneficial and harmful microbes, thus maintaining a balanced immune response.

4. Gut Barrier Integrity: The gut microbiome helps maintain the integrity of the gut barrier, which prevents harmful substances, toxins, and pathogens from entering the bloodstream.

5. Metabolism: Emerging research suggests that the gut microbiome can influence the host's metabolism, including energy balance, fat storage, and insulin sensitivity.

6. Neurotransmitter Production: Some gut bacteria can produce neurotransmitters and other bioactive compounds that can influence communication between the gut and the brain, forming the gut-brain axis.

7. Defense Against Pathogens: Beneficial gut bacteria can compete with and inhibit the growth of harmful pathogens, helping to protect the host from infections.

Impact of the Gut Microbiome on Health:

A balanced and diverse gut microbiome is associated with numerous health benefits, including:

- Improved digestion and nutrient absorption

- Enhanced immune function and reduced inflammation

- Protection against certain infections and diseases

- Better mental health and cognitive function

- Metabolic regulation and weight management support

- Reduced risk of certain chronic diseases, such as obesity, type 2 diabetes, and inflammatory bowel disease (IBD)

Conversely, an imbalance in the gut microbiome, known as dysbiosis, has been linked to various health conditions and diseases, including gastrointestinal disorders, autoimmune diseases, allergies, and mental health disorders.

In recent years, research into the gut microbiome has grown exponentially, revealing fascinating insights into its complex interactions with human health. Understanding the gut microbiome's significance opens up new avenues for personalized medicine and therapeutic interventions aimed at promoting gut health and overall well-being. As science continues to unravel the intricacies of the gut microbiome, it becomes increasingly evident that maintaining a healthy gut ecosystem is essential for optimizing health and preventing disease.

2.2 Role of Gut Microbes in Health

The gut microbiome plays a critical role in maintaining overall health and well-being. Its diverse community of microorganisms interacts with the host's body in multiple ways, influencing various physiological processes. Here are some key roles of gut microbes in health:

1. Digestion and Nutrient Metabolism: Gut microbes aid in the breakdown and fermentation of complex carbohydrates, fiber, and other compounds that human digestive enzymes cannot fully digest. This process produces short-chain fatty acids (SCFAs) and other beneficial metabolites, providing additional energy sources for the host and supporting gut health.

2. Immune System Regulation: The gut microbiome helps educate and regulate the immune system. Beneficial gut bacteria train the

immune system to recognize and tolerate harmless antigens while effectively responding to harmful pathogens. This immune education helps maintain a balanced and appropriate immune response.

3. Gut Barrier Integrity: Gut microbes play a crucial role in maintaining the integrity of the gut barrier. They contribute to the production of mucus and reinforce the gut lining, preventing the entry of harmful substances and pathogens into the bloodstream. A strong gut barrier is essential for overall health and immune function.

4. Production of Essential Nutrients: Some gut microbes produce vitamins (e.g., B vitamins and vitamin K) and other essential nutrients that are absorbed and

utilized by the host. This microbial contribution to nutrient production enhances the host's nutritional status.

5. Defense Against Pathogens: Beneficial gut bacteria help protect the host from harmful pathogens by competing for resources and producing antimicrobial substances. This defense mechanism helps prevent infections and keeps the gut ecosystem in balance.

6. Influence on Metabolism and Weight: Emerging research indicates that the gut microbiome can influence the host's metabolism, including energy balance and fat storage. An imbalance in the gut microbiome has been linked to obesity and metabolic disorders.

7. Gut-Brain Axis Communication: The gut microbiome communicates with the brain through the gut-brain axis. Gut microbes can produce neurotransmitters and other bioactive compounds that can influence mood, stress responses, and cognitive function.

8. Anti-Inflammatory Effects: Some gut microbes produce anti-inflammatory substances, helping to regulate inflammation in the gut and throughout the body. This anti-inflammatory activity contributes to overall health and may reduce the risk of inflammatory diseases.

9. Modulation of Disease Risk: The composition of the gut microbiome has been associated with the risk of various diseases, including

gastrointestinal disorders, autoimmune diseases, allergies, and mental health disorders.

10. Drug Metabolism: Gut microbes can influence the metabolism and efficacy of certain drugs, potentially impacting drug treatments and personalized medicine approaches.

Overall, the gut microbiome's roles are diverse and intertwined, and maintaining a healthy and balanced gut ecosystem is crucial for promoting overall health and preventing various diseases.

2.3 Difference between Probiotics and Prebiotics

Probiotics and prebiotics are both beneficial for gut health, but they are distinct substances with different functions.

Probiotics:

Probiotics are live microorganisms, primarily bacteria, that provide health benefits when consumed in adequate amounts. These beneficial bacteria can be found naturally in certain fermented foods, such as yogurt, kefir, sauerkraut, and kimchi. They can also be taken as supplements.

The key characteristics of probiotics are:

1. Live Organisms: Probiotics are living microorganisms that must be viable and survive the digestive process to reach the gut alive.

2. Beneficial Bacteria: Probiotics consist of specific strains of beneficial bacteria, such as

Lactobacillus and Bifidobacterium, which confer health benefits to the host.

3. Gut Microbiome Balance: Probiotics help maintain a balanced gut microbiome by supporting the growth of beneficial bacteria and inhibiting the growth of harmful ones.

4. Health Benefits: Probiotics have been associated with various health benefits, including improved digestion, enhanced immune function, reduced inflammation, and support for certain gastrointestinal conditions.

Prebiotics:

Prebiotics, on the other hand, are non-digestible fibers and compounds found in certain foods that serve as a food source for beneficial gut bacteria. They do not contain live microorganisms themselves but instead promote the growth and activity of probiotics and other beneficial microbes in the gut.

The key characteristics of prebiotics are:

1. Non-Living Compounds: Prebiotics are non-living substances that pass through the upper digestive tract intact and reach the colon, where they are fermented by beneficial gut bacteria.

2. Nourishment for Beneficial Bacteria: Prebiotics act as a substrate for the growth of specific strains of beneficial bacteria, particularly Bifidobacteria and Lactobacilli.

3. Gut Microbiome Support: By providing nourishment to beneficial bacteria, prebiotics help create a favorable gut environment and contribute to a diverse and thriving gut microbiome.

4. Health Benefits: Prebiotics have been associated with various health benefits, including improved gut health, enhanced nutrient absorption, immune system support, and potential effects on metabolic health.

Probiotics are live microorganisms that provide health benefits when ingested, while prebiotics are non-living compounds that nourish and promote the growth of beneficial gut bacteria. Combining probiotics and prebiotics in the diet is a strategy known as synbiotics, which aims to optimize gut health by providing both beneficial microorganisms and the food they need to thrive.

CHAPTER 3

Types of Prebiotic Foods

3.1 Inulin-Rich Foods

Inulin is a type of soluble fiber and a well-known prebiotic that is found in various plant-based foods. It consists of a chain of fructose molecules linked together, which the human digestive enzymes cannot break down. As a result, inulin reaches the colon largely intact, where it serves as a food source for beneficial gut bacteria, promoting their growth and activity. Here are some inulin-rich foods:

1. Chicory Root: Chicory root is one of the richest natural sources of

inulin. It is commonly used as a coffee substitute and is also used in various food products as a source of prebiotic fiber.

2. Jerusalem Artichoke: Also known as sunchokes, Jerusalem artichokes are tuberous vegetables that contain significant amounts of inulin.

3. Dandelion Greens: Dandelion greens are leafy greens that are rich in inulin and other nutrients. They can be used in salads or cooked as a vegetable.

4. Asparagus: Asparagus is a nutritious vegetable that contains inulin and is a great addition to various dishes.

5. Garlic: Garlic is not only a flavorful culinary ingredient but

also a source of inulin and other beneficial compounds.

6. Onions: Onions, particularly raw onions, are rich in inulin and can be used in salads, stir-fries, and various cooked dishes.

7. Leeks: Leeks belong to the onion family and are another source of inulin, commonly used in soups and stews.

8. Bananas: Unripe or green bananas contain resistant starch, which is a type of prebiotic. As bananas ripen, the resistant starch content decreases, but they still contain some inulin.

It is worth noting that some people may experience gastrointestinal discomfort when consuming large amounts of inulin-rich foods, as the fermentation of inulin by gut bacteria can lead to gas and bloating. Gradually increasing intake and consuming a variety of prebiotic foods can help minimize these side effects.

3.2 Fructooligosaccharides (FOS) Sources

Fructooligosaccharides (FOS) are another type of prebiotic fiber composed of short chains of fructose molecules. Like inulin, FOS is not fully digested in the upper gastrointestinal tract and reaches the colon intact, where it selectively feeds beneficial gut bacteria. Some common sources of FOS include:

1. Bananas: Ripe bananas contain
   FOS, in addition to inulin when
   they are unripe.

2. Blue Agave: Blue agave syrup,
   derived from the agave plant, is a
   natural sweetener that contains
   FOS.

3. Jicama: Jicama is a crunchy root
   vegetable that provides FOS and
   can be enjoyed raw or cooked.

4. Asparagus: Along with containing
   inulin, asparagus is a source of
   FOS.

5. Wheat: Wheat-based products,
   such as wheat bran and certain
   whole-grain foods, contain FOS.

6. Barley: Barley is a grain that
   contains FOS and other prebiotic
   fibers.

7. Artichokes: Globe artichokes are a
source of FOS and can be cooked
and enjoyed as a tasty vegetable.

8. Honey: Raw honey contains small
amounts of FOS, contributing to
its prebiotic properties.

It's important to note that FOS is
commonly used as a functional
ingredient in some food products and
supplements to increase their
prebiotic content. As with inulin,
gradually incorporating FOS-rich
foods into the diet can help
individuals adapt to the increased
fiber intake and reduce the likelihood
of digestive discomfort.

Consuming a diverse range of
prebiotic foods, including those rich
in inulin and FOS, can contribute to a
healthy gut microbiome and support
overall gut health. Additionally,

combining prebiotic-rich foods with probiotics in the diet can create a synergistic effect, optimizing the benefits for gut health.

3.3 Galactooligosaccharides (GOS) Sources

Galactooligosaccharides (GOS) are a type of prebiotic fiber composed of short chains of galactose molecules. Similar to other prebiotics, GOS reaches the colon undigested, where it serves as a food source for beneficial gut bacteria, particularly Bifidobacteria. GOS is often found in human breast milk, providing nourishment to the gut microbiome of infants. Additionally, GOS is used as an ingredient in some infant formulas to mimic the prebiotic benefits of breast milk. Here are some sources of GOS:

1. Human Breast Milk: Human breast milk is naturally rich in GOS and provides essential nourishment for newborns.

2. Infant Formulas: Some infant formulas are supplemented with GOS to support the growth of beneficial gut bacteria in formula-fed babies.

3. Legumes: Certain legumes, such as chickpeas and lentils, contain GOS and can be included in the diet.

4. Cow's Milk: Cow's milk also contains small amounts of GOS, but its concentration is significantly lower than that of human breast milk.

5. Nuts: Nuts, particularly almonds, contain GOS and can be incorporated into the diet for added prebiotic benefits.

6. Soy Products: Some soy-based foods, like soy milk and tofu, contain GOS.

7. Certain Grains: Grains like wheat and rye can contain GOS, contributing to their prebiotic properties.

8. GOS Supplements: GOS supplements are available and can be used to increase prebiotic intake when dietary sources are limited.

GOS provides specific benefits to the gut microbiome, particularly in supporting the growth and activity of Bifidobacteria, which are considered beneficial for gut health.

3.4 Resistant Starch Foods

Resistant starch is a type of starch that resists digestion in the small intestine and reaches the colon intact, where it serves as a prebiotic fiber for beneficial gut bacteria. Resistant starch comes in different types, with each having different effects on gut health. Some common sources of resistant starch include:

1. Green Bananas: Unripe or green bananas are a significant source of resistant starch. As bananas ripen, the resistant starch content decreases.

2. Cooked and Cooled Potatoes: When cooked and then cooled, potatoes undergo a process called retrogradation, which increases the formation of resistant starch.

3. Legumes: Beans, lentils, and peas
    are excellent sources of resistant
    starch.

4. Whole Grains: Some whole grains,
    such as oats and barley, contain
    resistant starch.

5. Cold Pasta and Rice: When pasta
    or rice is cooked and then cooled,
    it becomes a source of resistant
    starch.

6. Corn: Corn contains a type of
    resistant starch that is beneficial
    for gut health.

Resistant starch provides various
health benefits, including promoting
the growth of beneficial gut bacteria,
improving insulin sensitivity, and
supporting digestive health.

3.5 Other Natural Prebiotic Sources

In addition to inulin, FOS, GOS, and resistant starch, several other natural foods contain prebiotic properties. Some of these include:

1. Apples: Apples contain pectin, a type of prebiotic fiber that supports gut health.

2. Cocoa: Cocoa and dark chocolate contain polyphenols, which can act as prebiotics and support gut health.

3. Flaxseeds: Flaxseeds are a source of prebiotic fibers and omega-3 fatty acids.

4. Seaweed: Certain types of seaweed, like kelp and nori, contain prebiotic compounds.

5. Dried Fruits: Dried fruits like figs, dates, and raisins provide prebiotic benefits.

6. Yacon Root: Yacon root is rich in fructooligosaccharides (FOS), making it a natural prebiotic source.

7. Burdock Root: Burdock root contains inulin, contributing to its prebiotic properties.

8. Konjac Root: Konjac root is high in glucomannan, a type of prebiotic fiber.

9. Greens: Leafy greens, such as spinach and kale, contain fiber that can act as prebiotics.

10. Berries: Berries, like raspberries and blackberries, contain fiber that supports gut health.

Including a variety of these natural prebiotic sources in the diet can help promote a diverse and thriving gut microbiome, contributing to better gut health and overall well-being. As with any dietary change, it's essential to gradually introduce prebiotic-rich foods and monitor individual responses.

CHAPTER 4

Health Benefits of Prebiotics

4.1 Improved Digestive Health

Prebiotics play a vital role in promoting improved digestive health by supporting the growth and activity of beneficial gut bacteria. When prebiotic fibers reach the colon undigested, they serve as a food source for these beneficial microbes, particularly Bifidobacteria and Lactobacilli. The fermentation of prebiotics by these bacteria produces short-chain fatty acids (SCFAs), such as butyrate, acetate, and propionate, which have several positive effects on the digestive system:

1. Enhanced Gut Barrier Function: SCFAs help strengthen the gut barrier by promoting the production of mucus and reinforcing the intestinal lining. A strong gut barrier helps prevent the entry of harmful substances and pathogens into the bloodstream, reducing the risk of gut-related infections and inflammation.

2. Reduced Risk of Gastrointestinal Disorders: Prebiotics contribute to a balanced gut microbiome, which is associated with a reduced risk of gastrointestinal disorders such as irritable bowel syndrome (IBS), inflammatory bowel disease (IBD), and constipation.

3. Improved Bowel Regularity:
   Consuming prebiotic-rich foods
   can promote bowel regularity and
   alleviate symptoms of constipation
   by supporting healthy gut motility.

4. Reduced Gastrointestinal
   Inflammation: SCFAs have anti-
   inflammatory properties and can
   help regulate inflammation in the
   gut, providing relief to individuals
   with inflammatory conditions like
   ulcerative colitis and Crohn's
   disease.

5. Minimized Gastrointestinal
   Discomfort: Beneficial gut bacteria
   break down prebiotics in a
   controlled manner, reducing
   excessive gas production and
   bloating often associated with the
   fermentation of other poorly
   digestible fibers.

Overall, the presence of prebiotics in the diet supports a healthier gut environment, which positively influences digestive health and helps prevent and manage various gastrointestinal issues.

4.2 Enhanced Nutrient Absorption

A healthy and diverse gut microbiome, supported by prebiotics, can enhance nutrient absorption and utilization in several ways:

1. Improved Calcium Absorption: Prebiotics, particularly inulin-type fructans, have been shown to improve calcium absorption in the gut. This can be beneficial for maintaining bone health and reducing the risk of osteoporosis.

2. Increased Magnesium Absorption:
    Prebiotics can enhance the
    absorption of magnesium, an
    essential mineral involved in
    various physiological processes,
    including nerve function, muscle
    contraction, and energy
    production.

3. Enhanced Iron Bioavailability:
    Prebiotics can increase the
    bioavailability of iron from plant-
    based sources, making it easier for
    the body to absorb and utilize this
    important mineral.

4. Support for B-Vitamin Production:
    Beneficial gut bacteria fed by
    prebiotics can produce certain B-
    vitamins, such as biotin and folate,
    which contribute to various bodily
    functions, including energy
    metabolism and DNA synthesis.

5. Enhanced Short-Chain Fatty Acid Production: SCFAs, derived from prebiotic fermentation, not only benefit the gut but also support overall health. For instance, butyrate has been associated with improved colon health and may even have anti-cancer effects.

By promoting the growth of beneficial gut bacteria and enhancing the production of SCFAs, prebiotics create an optimal gut environment for improved nutrient absorption and utilization. As a result, individuals who regularly consume prebiotic-rich foods may experience increased overall nutrient uptake and better overall nutritional status.

It is important to note that while prebiotics can enhance nutrient absorption and digestive health, individual responses may vary.

Factors such as gut microbiome composition, gut health, and underlying medical conditions can influence the extent of these benefits. Nevertheless, incorporating prebiotic-rich foods into a balanced diet can be a valuable strategy to support digestive health and optimize nutrient absorption.

4.3 Immune System Support

The gut microbiome plays a significant role in supporting the immune system, and prebiotics contribute to immune system support by promoting a healthy and balanced gut ecosystem. Beneficial gut bacteria, which are nourished by prebiotics, interact with the immune system in several ways:

1. Modulation of Immune Responses:
   Prebiotics help regulate the
   immune system, promoting a
   balanced and appropriate response.
   They stimulate the production of
   anti-inflammatory cytokines while
   reducing the production of pro-
   inflammatory cytokines, creating a
   harmonious immune environment.

2. Enhanced Gut-Associated
   Lymphoid Tissue (GALT)
   Function: The gut-associated
   lymphoid tissue (GALT) is a
   significant component of the
   immune system located in the gut.
   The presence of prebiotics in the
   diet helps maintain the health and
   function of GALT, supporting its
   role in immune surveillance and
   response.

3. Improved Barrier Function: A
   healthy gut barrier is essential for

immune system support, as it prevents harmful substances and pathogens from crossing into the bloodstream. Prebiotics contribute to the production of mucus and the reinforcement of the gut lining, enhancing the barrier's integrity.

4. Protection Against Pathogens: Beneficial gut bacteria, fueled by prebiotics, compete with harmful pathogens for nutrients and colonization sites. This competitive exclusion helps protect against infections and supports the body's defense mechanisms.

Overall, by promoting a balanced and diverse gut microbiome, prebiotics play a vital role in supporting the immune system and reducing the risk of immune-related disorders and infections.

4.4 Weight Management and Prebiotics

Prebiotics may play a role in weight management and metabolic health due to their influence on the gut microbiome and overall gut health. Some ways in which prebiotics can contribute to weight management include:

1. Increased Satiety: Prebiotics, particularly certain types of fiber, can increase feelings of fullness and satiety after meals. This may help reduce overall calorie intake and support weight management efforts.

2. Regulation of Appetite Hormones: Prebiotics can influence the production of appetite-regulating hormones, such as ghrelin and

peptide YY (PYY), helping to regulate hunger and appetite.

3. Impact on Energy Metabolism: Prebiotics, especially resistant starch, may influence energy metabolism, affecting how the body processes and stores energy from food.

4. Reduction of Adiposity: Some studies suggest that prebiotics can lead to a reduction in adiposity (body fat) by promoting beneficial changes in gut bacteria and metabolic pathways.

5. Improved Insulin Sensitivity: Prebiotics have been associated with improved insulin sensitivity, which can positively impact blood sugar levels and reduce the risk of type 2 diabetes and metabolic syndrome.

It is essential to recognize that while prebiotics can contribute to weight management, they are not a standalone solution for weight loss. A balanced diet, regular physical activity, and overall lifestyle choices are crucial for achieving and maintaining a healthy weight.

4.5 Mental Health and Prebiotics

Emerging research indicates that there is a connection between gut health and mental health, commonly referred to as the gut-brain axis. Prebiotics play a role in this connection by influencing the gut microbiome and the production of neurotransmitters. Here's how prebiotics may contribute to mental health:

1. Gut-Brain Communication: The gut and brain communicate through neural, hormonal, and immune pathways. Prebiotics can influence this communication by supporting the gut microbiome, which produces various neuroactive compounds and neurotransmitters that affect brain function.

2. Production of Neurotransmitters: Some beneficial gut bacteria can produce neurotransmitters like serotonin and gamma-aminobutyric acid (GABA). These neurotransmitters play essential roles in mood regulation and anxiety reduction.

3. Anti-Inflammatory Effects: Prebiotics' anti-inflammatory properties can positively impact brain health, as inflammation has

been linked to various mental health disorders.

4. Stress Regulation: The gut microbiome can influence the body's response to stress, and prebiotics may play a role in modulating the stress response.

While more research is needed to fully understand the impact of prebiotics on mental health, the gut-brain axis is a fascinating area of study with promising implications for mental health interventions. In addition to prebiotics, a balanced diet, regular exercise, adequate sleep, and stress management are essential components of a holistic approach to mental well-being.

Prebiotics support various aspects of health, including immune system function, weight management, and potential implications for mental health. By promoting a diverse and balanced gut microbiome, prebiotics contribute to overall wellness and may reduce the risk of certain diseases and health conditions. As with any dietary change, it is essential to consult with a healthcare professional before making significant modifications to one's diet.

CHAPTER 5

Incorporating Prebiotics into Your Diet

5.1 Gradual Dietary Changes

When incorporating prebiotics into your diet, it is essential to make gradual dietary changes to allow your gut microbiome to adapt slowly. Rapidly increasing your prebiotic intake can lead to gastrointestinal discomfort, such as gas and bloating, especially if you are not accustomed to consuming significant amounts of fiber. Here are some tips for making gradual dietary changes:

1. Start with Small Portions: Begin by adding small portions of prebiotic-rich foods to your meals. For example, start with half a serving of a prebiotic vegetable or legume and gradually increase the amount over time.

2. Monitor Your Body's Response: Pay attention to how your body responds to the increased fiber intake. If you experience mild digestive discomfort, reduce the portion size and increase it gradually once your body adapts.

3. Diversify Prebiotic Sources: Include a variety of prebiotic-rich foods in your diet to promote a diverse gut microbiome. Rotate different sources of prebiotics to provide a wide range of beneficial fibers.

4. Stay Hydrated: Drinking plenty of water is essential when increasing your fiber intake. Water helps move fiber through the digestive system and can alleviate some digestive discomfort.

5. Consider Prebiotic Supplements: If you find it challenging to incorporate enough prebiotics through diet alone, consider adding a prebiotic supplement to your routine. However, it is always best to obtain nutrients from whole foods whenever possible.

5.2 Recommended Daily Intake

There is no specific recommended daily intake for prebiotics like there is for essential nutrients. The amount of prebiotics needed varies based on factors such as age, sex, body size, and individual health goals. However, dietary guidelines generally recommend a daily fiber intake for adults of around 25 to 38 grams, depending on gender and age.

When it comes to prebiotic-rich foods, there is no strict limit to how much you can consume. Instead, focus on incorporating a variety of prebiotic sources into your diet to promote a diverse gut microbiome. Aim to include prebiotic foods in most meals and snacks to support gut health regularly.

5.3 Cooking and Prebiotic Foods

Cooking can impact the prebiotic content of foods, but there are ways to preserve prebiotic properties while preparing meals:

1. Raw Consumption: Some prebiotic-rich foods are best consumed raw to retain their full prebiotic potential. For example, raw garlic and raw onions are excellent prebiotic choices.

2. Light Cooking: Lightly cooking prebiotic vegetables, such as asparagus and leeks, can soften them without fully degrading the prebiotic fibers.

3. Cooling and Retrogradation: Certain foods, like cooked potatoes and pasta, can form resistant starch

and become prebiotic when cooled. Consider eating them in salads or after refrigeration.

4. Steam Instead of Boil: Steaming vegetables instead of boiling them can help retain more of their prebiotic fiber content.

5. Avoid Overcooking: Overcooking prebiotic-rich foods can break down their fiber content and reduce their prebiotic properties. Cook them until they are just tender.

6. Combine with Probiotics: Combining prebiotic-rich foods with probiotic-rich foods (such as fermented foods like yogurt) can create a synergistic effect, optimizing the benefits for gut health.

Remember that each person's tolerance to prebiotic foods can vary, so it's essential to find a balance that works for your body. If you have specific health concerns or medical conditions, consult with a healthcare professional or registered dietitian for personalized dietary recommendations.

Incorporating prebiotic-rich foods into your diet can be a valuable step towards supporting gut health and overall well-being. By making gradual changes and consuming a variety of prebiotic sources, you can nurture a diverse and thriving gut microbiome that contributes to better digestion, improved immune function, and potential benefits for other aspects of health.

5.4 Potential Side Effects and How to Minimize Them

While prebiotics offer numerous health benefits, some individuals may experience side effects, especially when significantly increasing their prebiotic intake. Common side effects include gas, bloating, abdominal discomfort, and changes in bowel movements. These side effects are often temporary and can be minimized with some strategies:

1. Gradual Increase: As mentioned earlier, gradually increase your prebiotic intake to allow your gut microbiome to adapt slowly. Start with small portions of prebiotic-rich foods and gradually increase the amount over time.

2. Diversify Prebiotic Sources:
   Consume a variety of prebiotic-
   rich foods rather than focusing on
   a single source. Diversifying your
   prebiotic intake can reduce the risk
   of excessive fermentation of a
   specific fiber type, which may
   contribute to digestive discomfort.

3. Cook and Prepare Foods Wisely:
   Lightly cook prebiotic vegetables
   and avoid overcooking to preserve
   their prebiotic fiber content.
   Incorporate raw or lightly cooked
   options to maintain their prebiotic
   potential.

4. Stay Hydrated: Drinking plenty of
   water can help move fiber through
   the digestive system and alleviate
   some digestive discomfort
   associated with increased prebiotic
   intake.

5. Monitor Portion Sizes: Pay
    attention to portion sizes of
    prebiotic foods, especially if you
    are sensitive to certain fibers.
    Adjust portion sizes as needed
    based on your individual tolerance.

6. Combine with Probiotics:
    Consuming prebiotic-rich foods
    with probiotic-rich foods can
    create a balanced gut environment
    and may help reduce potential side
    effects.

7. Probiotic Supplements: If you
    experience digestive discomfort
    with prebiotic consumption, you
    may consider taking probiotic
    supplements alongside prebiotics.
    Probiotics can help balance gut
    bacteria and alleviate some
    digestive issues.

8. Prebiotic Supplements: If you struggle to get enough prebiotics from dietary sources or need a more controlled approach, consider taking prebiotic supplements. However, consult with a healthcare professional before starting any supplement regimen.

9. Monitor and Adjust: Keep track of how your body responds to prebiotic consumption. If you experience persistent or severe discomfort, consider reducing your prebiotic intake or consulting with a healthcare professional.

It's essential to recognize that everyone's gut microbiome is unique, and individual responses to prebiotics can vary. What works well for one person may not be suitable for another. It's crucial to listen to your body, make adjustments as needed, and prioritize a balanced diet that supports overall health.

If you have specific health conditions or concerns, or if you experience persistent or severe gastrointestinal symptoms, consult with a healthcare professional or a registered dietitian. They can provide personalized recommendations and guidance to optimize your gut health and overall well-being.

CHAPTER 6

Prebiotics and Special Health Conditions

6.1 Prebiotics for Irritable Bowel Syndrome (IBS)

Irritable Bowel Syndrome (IBS) is a common gastrointestinal disorder characterized by abdominal pain, bloating, and changes in bowel habits, such as diarrhea, constipation, or both. While the exact cause of IBS is not fully understood, it is believed to involve disturbances in gut motility, sensitivity, and the gut-brain axis.

Prebiotics can potentially offer benefits for individuals with IBS due to their effects on gut health and the gut microbiome. However, the response to prebiotics can vary among individuals with IBS, and some people may experience worsened symptoms if they are sensitive to certain fibers. Here are some considerations for using prebiotics for IBS:

1. Low-FODMAP Approach: The FODMAP diet is an effective dietary approach for managing IBS symptoms. FODMAPs are fermentable carbohydrates that can trigger digestive symptoms in some individuals with IBS. While some prebiotic foods are high in FODMAPs (e.g., onions, garlic, and certain legumes), others are

low in FODMAPs and may be better tolerated.

2. Gradual Introduction: If considering prebiotic consumption, introduce them gradually and in small amounts to gauge your individual tolerance. Some prebiotics, such as inulin and fructooligosaccharides (FOS), may worsen symptoms in some individuals with IBS.

3. Individual Sensitivity: Monitor how your body responds to different types of prebiotics. Some individuals with IBS may find that certain prebiotics exacerbate symptoms, while others may be well-tolerated.

4. Consult a Healthcare Professional: If you have IBS or digestive concerns, it is essential to work

with a healthcare professional or a registered dietitian to develop a personalized dietary plan. They can help you identify trigger foods, recommend suitable prebiotic sources, and guide you on balancing your gut health.

6.2 Prebiotics and Diabetes Management

Diabetes is a metabolic disorder characterized by high blood sugar levels resulting from either insufficient insulin production (Type 1 diabetes) or insulin resistance (Type 2 diabetes). Managing blood sugar levels is critical for diabetes management, and prebiotics may play a role in supporting overall health and glucose regulation. Here's how prebiotics may impact diabetes management:

1. Improved Insulin Sensitivity: Prebiotics have been associated with improved insulin sensitivity, meaning that the body's cells become more responsive to insulin, facilitating glucose uptake and utilization.

2. Reduced Postprandial Glucose Spikes: Prebiotics, particularly resistant starch, can slow down the digestion and absorption of carbohydrates, leading to more gradual and stable rises in blood sugar levels after meals.

3. Weight Management: Prebiotics may contribute to weight management by increasing feelings of fullness and reducing overall calorie intake. Maintaining a

healthy weight is essential for diabetes management.

4. Reduced Inflammation: Some prebiotics have anti-inflammatory properties, and reducing inflammation may benefit individuals with diabetes, as chronic inflammation is associated with insulin resistance.

It is important to note that prebiotics are not a replacement for standard diabetes management, which includes medication (if necessary), blood sugar monitoring, a balanced diet, and regular physical activity. Individuals with diabetes should work with their healthcare team to develop a comprehensive diabetes management plan that considers their specific health needs.

As with any dietary change, consult with a healthcare professional or a registered dietitian before incorporating prebiotics or making significant modifications to your diet, especially if you have special health conditions or medical concerns. They can provide personalized guidance to help you optimize your gut health while considering your individual health needs.

6.3 Prebiotics and Heart Health

Prebiotics may play a role in promoting heart health through their effects on the gut microbiome and overall gut health. Several mechanisms suggest how prebiotics may benefit cardiovascular health:

1. Cholesterol Management: Some prebiotics, particularly certain types of soluble fiber like beta-glucans and psyllium, have been shown to help reduce LDL cholesterol levels (the "bad" cholesterol) by interfering with cholesterol absorption in the gut.

2. Blood Pressure Regulation: Prebiotics may contribute to blood pressure regulation by promoting a healthy gut microbiome, which can have indirect effects on blood pressure through various pathways.

3. Anti-Inflammatory Effects: Chronic inflammation is a risk factor for cardiovascular disease. Prebiotics' anti-inflammatory properties, particularly the production of short-chain fatty acids (SCFAs), may help reduce

inflammation in the body,
including the cardiovascular
system.

4. Weight Management: Maintaining
   a healthy weight is crucial for
   heart health. Prebiotics can
   increase feelings of fullness and
   satiety, which may help with
   weight management and reduce
   the risk of obesity-related
   cardiovascular risk factors.

5. Insulin Sensitivity: Improved
   insulin sensitivity, supported by
   prebiotics, may have positive
   effects on metabolic health, which
   is linked to heart health.

While prebiotics can be part of a
heart-healthy lifestyle, it's important
to remember that heart health is
influenced by various factors,
including a balanced diet, regular

physical activity, not smoking, managing stress, and maintaining a healthy weight. A comprehensive approach to heart health is essential, and individuals should consult with their healthcare provider or a registered dietitian to develop a personalized plan.

6.4 Prebiotics for Immune-Related Disorders

The relationship between the gut microbiome and the immune system is significant, and prebiotics may have implications for immune-related disorders. While research in this area is still evolving, prebiotics' effects on the gut microbiome can influence immune function in several ways:

1. Modulation of Immune Responses:
   Prebiotics can help regulate the
   immune system, promoting a
   balanced response and reducing
   the risk of immune-related
   disorders characterized by
   excessive or inappropriate immune
   activation.

2. Enhanced Gut-Associated
   Lymphoid Tissue (GALT)
   Function: The gut-associated
   lymphoid tissue (GALT) is a
   crucial component of the immune
   system located in the gut.
   Prebiotics can support GALT
   function, contributing to improved
   immune surveillance and response.

3. Protection Against Pathogens:
   Beneficial gut bacteria, supported
   by prebiotics, can compete with
   harmful pathogens for nutrients
   and colonization sites, helping to

protect against infections and support the body's defense mechanisms.

4. Reduced Inflammation: Prebiotics' anti-inflammatory effects can positively impact immune health, as chronic inflammation is linked to various immune-related disorders.

5. Impact on Autoimmune Conditions: The gut microbiome may influence the development and progression of autoimmune conditions. While more research is needed, prebiotics may potentially have implications for managing certain autoimmune disorders.

It's important to note that the effects of prebiotics on immune-related disorders can vary among individuals, and more research is needed to fully understand their impact on specific conditions. If you have an immune-related disorder or are considering using prebiotics for immune support, consult with a healthcare professional to discuss the potential benefits and risks in your specific case.

Overall, prebiotics have the potential to influence heart health and immune function positively. However, as with any health condition, individual responses can vary, and it's essential to work with healthcare professionals to develop a comprehensive and personalized approach to managing heart health and immune-related concerns.

CHAPTER 7

Best Practices for Prebiotic Health

7.1 Balancing Prebiotics and Probiotics

Balancing prebiotics and probiotics in your diet can optimize gut health and support a diverse and thriving gut microbiome. Prebiotics and probiotics work together to create a synergistic effect, promoting beneficial changes in the gut ecosystem. Here are some best practices for balancing prebiotics and probiotics:

1. Include a Variety of Prebiotic Foods: Consume a diverse range of prebiotic-rich foods, such as

vegetables, fruits, whole grains,
and legumes. Aim to have a mix of
inulin, FOS, GOS, and resistant
starch sources to support different
types of beneficial gut bacteria.

2. Incorporate Probiotic-Rich Foods:
    Consume probiotic-rich foods
    regularly, such as yogurt, kefir,
    sauerkraut, kimchi, and other
    fermented foods. These foods
    introduce live beneficial bacteria
    to the gut.

3. Consider Prebiotic Supplements: If
    it's challenging to obtain sufficient
    prebiotics from dietary sources,
    consider adding a prebiotic
    supplement to your routine. This
    can complement the probiotics you
    consume and support their growth
    and activity.

4. Time Your Consumption:
    Consider the timing of consuming
    prebiotic and probiotic foods.
    Consuming them together can
    create a more favorable
    environment for the beneficial
    bacteria to thrive.

5. Gradually Introduce: If you are
    new to consuming prebiotic or
    probiotic-rich foods, introduce
    them gradually to allow your gut
    microbiome to adapt slowly.

6. Pay Attention to Your Body:
    Listen to your body's response to
    prebiotic and probiotic
    consumption. If you experience
    any discomfort or unusual
    symptoms, adjust your intake
    accordingly.

7.2 Prebiotics and Antibiotics

Antibiotics are medications used to treat bacterial infections, but they can also disrupt the balance of beneficial gut bacteria along with harmful bacteria. This can lead to digestive issues and potential infections. Prebiotics can play a role in supporting gut health during and after antibiotic use. Here are some best practices for incorporating prebiotics during antibiotic therapy:

1. Timing Matters: Avoid taking prebiotic supplements or consuming prebiotic-rich foods at the same time as antibiotics. Give your body some time (ideally a few hours) between taking antibiotics and consuming prebiotics.

2. Complete the Full Antibiotic Course: Always finish the full course of antibiotics prescribed by your healthcare professional to effectively treat the infection and reduce the risk of antibiotic resistance.

3. Focus on Resistant Starch: During antibiotic use, focus on consuming more resistant starch, found in green bananas, cold pasta, and cooked and cooled potatoes. Resistant starch is less fermentable than other prebiotics and may be better tolerated during antibiotic treatment.

4. Replenish Beneficial Bacteria: After completing the antibiotic course, consider increasing your consumption of prebiotics and probiotics to help replenish beneficial gut bacteria.

5. Consider Probiotic Supplements: During and after antibiotic treatment, consider taking probiotic supplements to help maintain gut health. Choose supplements that contain a variety of beneficial bacterial strains.

6. Work with a Healthcare Professional: If you have concerns about antibiotic use and its impact on gut health, consult with your healthcare professional or a registered dietitian. They can provide personalized advice and recommendations based on your health status.

Remember that while prebiotics and probiotics can support gut health, they are not a substitute for medical treatment. Always follow your healthcare professional's advice regarding the use of antibiotics and any other medications.

Incorporating prebiotic-rich foods and probiotics into your diet can contribute to a healthy gut microbiome and overall well-being. By following these best practices, you can optimize your prebiotic health and promote a balanced and thriving gut ecosystem.

7.3 Lifestyle Factors for Gut Health

Maintaining a healthy gut goes beyond just consuming prebiotics and probiotics. Several lifestyle factors play a crucial role in supporting gut health and promoting a diverse gut microbiome. Here are some key lifestyle factors to consider:

1. Balanced Diet: Consume a balanced and varied diet rich in fiber from fruits, vegetables, whole grains, and legumes. Include prebiotic-rich foods to nourish beneficial gut bacteria and probiotic-rich foods to introduce live beneficial bacteria.

2. Regular Physical Activity: Engage in regular exercise, as it has been associated with a more diverse gut microbiome and improved gut health. Exercise can positively influence gut motility and microbial composition.

3. Adequate Sleep: Prioritize getting enough quality sleep each night, as poor sleep patterns can negatively affect gut health and disrupt the gut microbiome.

4. Reduce Stress: Chronic stress can impact gut health and alter the gut-brain axis. Incorporate stress-reducing practices like meditation, yoga, deep breathing, or spending time in nature.

5. Avoid Smoking and Excessive Alcohol: Smoking and excessive alcohol consumption can disrupt the gut microbiome and negatively affect gut health. Minimize or avoid these habits to support a healthy gut.

6. Limit Use of Antibiotics: Overuse of antibiotics can disrupt the gut microbiome. Only use antibiotics when necessary and as prescribed by your healthcare professional.

7. Avoid Unnecessary Use of Antimicrobial Products: Excessive use of antimicrobial products like

hand sanitizers and antibacterial soaps can disrupt the balance of beneficial gut bacteria. Use them sparingly and opt for regular soap and water when possible.

8. Stay Hydrated: Proper hydration supports digestion and helps move fiber through the digestive system. Drink plenty of water throughout the day.

7.4 Importance of Hydration

Hydration is essential for overall health, including gut health. Proper hydration helps maintain digestive function and supports a healthy gut microbiome. Here's why hydration is important for gut health:

1. Promotes Regular Bowel
   Movements: Drinking enough
   water helps soften stools and
   promotes regular bowel
   movements, preventing
   constipation and supporting gut
   motility.

2. Aids in Nutrient Absorption:
   Water plays a role in breaking
   down and absorbing nutrients from
   food, which is vital for overall
   health and optimal gut function.

3. Supports Beneficial Bacteria:
   Adequate hydration creates an
   optimal environment for beneficial
   gut bacteria to thrive, supporting a
   diverse and balanced gut
   microbiome.

4. Prevents Dehydration:
   Dehydration can lead to
   constipation and other digestive

issues. Ensuring adequate
hydration helps prevent these
problems.

5. Supports Gut Barrier Function:
    Hydration helps maintain the
    integrity of the gut lining,
    supporting the gut barrier's
    function and preventing harmful
    substances from entering the
    bloodstream.

To stay properly hydrated, aim to
drink at least eight 8-ounce glasses of
water per day, or more if you are
physically active or live in a hot
climate. Keep in mind that individual
hydration needs can vary based on
age, activity level, and other factors.

7.5 Stress Management and Gut Health

The gut-brain axis is a bidirectional communication system between the gut and the brain, and stress can significantly impact gut health. Chronic stress can disrupt the gut microbiome and lead to gastrointestinal issues. Here's how stress management can positively influence gut health:

1. Reduced Inflammation: Chronic stress can lead to increased inflammation, which is associated with gut issues. Stress management practices can help reduce inflammation and support gut health.

2. Balanced Gut Microbiome: Stress can alter the composition of the gut microbiome. Managing stress

can help promote a diverse and balanced gut microbiome, which is essential for gut health.

3. Improved Gut Motility: Stress can affect gut motility, leading to symptoms like diarrhea or constipation. Stress management practices can help regulate gut motility.

4. Enhanced Gut Barrier Function: Stress can compromise the gut barrier function, increasing the risk of gut-related issues. Managing stress supports a healthy gut lining and gut barrier.

Stress management practices can include meditation, deep breathing exercises, yoga, spending time in nature, engaging in hobbies, and seeking social support. Regular exercise and adequate sleep are also important components of stress management. By prioritizing stress management, you can positively influence your gut health and overall well-being.

a combination of prebiotic-rich foods, probiotics, and healthy lifestyle practices is essential for promoting gut health. By considering these best practices, you can support a diverse and balanced gut microbiome, which is crucial for digestive health, immune function, and overall wellness. Always consult with a healthcare professional or a registered dietitian for personalized advice based on your individual health needs and conditions.

www.ingramcontent.com/pod-product-compliance
Lightning Source LLC
Chambersburg PA
CBHW070954250726
48663CB00002B/214